Chapter 1- Introduction:

Fitness is a word that has been more abused than fast food over the last ten years. It seems like every day there is a new YouTube fitness sensation or infomercial channel trying to sell you something that will make you fit quickly and with minimal effort. I Google searched 'ab cruncher' so I could provide an example here. I was not surprised to see pictures of six different pieces of equipment, all claiming quick and easy results for a more chiseled physique. There is no single solution to achieving full body fitness and I'm sick of hearing liars claiming the contrary. I'm also sick of overweight, cigarette smoking doctors preaching the importance of good health to everybody that walks into their office. I've only seen two healthy looking doctors in my life and that seems quite ironic to me.

The broad definition of fitness is: 'the condition of being physically fit and healthy' but we need to get more specific for the purpose of this book. I once said "I'd rather be moderately fit, than extremely strong" and I still stand beside that statement, even though most of my friends thought it was stupid. As a 23 year old male, discrediting strength in any way is a surefire way to look weak in front of other guys. The truth of the matter is that strength is only one of many dimensions of fitness. By being a well-rounded fit person, strength is implied. Would you rather eat a big plate full of only steak, or have a modest portion of steak and indulge in the rest of the buffet?

I define fitness as a 'general sense of well being stemming from a multitude of different factors including, but not limited to, physical activeness, body image, coordination, diet, sleep schedule and mental stimulation.' This sounds like a lot and it is, which is why increasing fitness takes way more than a piece of workout equipment, a five minute per day circuit, or some kind of 'super supplement. This is lesson number one: fitness is not an easy thing to achieve; it is something that you should strive for. If it were easy there would be a lot more fit people, but it takes consistent effort and it is this effort that makes it worth it in the end.

As I write this I am on a two-month road trip around the United States and I feel awful, even though I'm having an amazing time with fantastic people. Why do I feel awful you ask? Because my fitness level has decreased dramatically since I left Canada. When you leave your regular life and restrict yourself to the confines of a small vehicle, it becomes relatively easy to isolate factors that are affecting your personal happiness. My physical activity has plummeted, my flexibility has gone down the drain, my diet consists of mostly canned food and my sleep schedule is a train wreck. Before I willingly crammed myself into this small Mitsubishi, I felt amazing. I was active every day, eating well, sleeping well and having lots of sex.

Fitness should not be viewed as a quick fad, or a state that you can achieve and then have forever. It is a lifestyle that needs to be maintained regularly- just like a car. Don't let yourself become one of those people who care more about what they're putting in their car, than what they're putting in their own bodies, or you're sure to break down regularly. Think about it; your body is an extremely complex machine. If you're not particular about how you're fueling it and how you're running it, then you are destined to crash and burn.

My name is John Mayo, I'm not very flexible, my sleep patterns vary, I eat horrible food a couple times a week, drink alcohol on occasion, have sex as much as possible and I consider myself fairly fit. I'm not writing this in an attempt to stroke my ego; I'm just an average guy who likes to feel good as much as I can. I got into fitness at a young age as a flat-water kayaker and experienced success in the sport for the seven years that I competed. I became a national champion in two events and got to travel to the United States and Europe to compete.

When I quit kayaking due to a back injury I became very paranoid about falling out of shape. This paranoia originated from the fact that I was going from a structured daily training regiment, to absolutely nothing.

Sport and fitness were all I had known growing up, so once university started I began hitting the gym solo for the first time in my life. I began to practice Brazilian jiu jitsu and I started developing my own workout plans, which I really began to enjoy. I liked the idea of engineering my own fitness, stretching my physical limits and being able to push myself without a coach. Four years ago I ran a marathon on my own, just to see if I could mentally and physically force myself to do so.

Modern life seems to trick our minds into thinking that, we should behave in a certain way; sleep eight hours, work eight hours, eat when we can, have sex when we can, try to raise a family and repeat. This is the cycle that traps many people and before they know it they are unhappy with their lives, likely due to the fact that they are unhappy with themselves. Just because our species has evolved in exponential ways over a brief period of time, doesn't mean we can forget our roots and genetics.

Our species survival is due to our rapid evolution of intelligence and fitness. Remember, it's survival of the fittest, not the mere existence of the complacent. We are at the top of the food chain because we have the physical abilities to act upon our ideas.

It's a well-known fact that human beings are the best long distance runners on planet earth. Yes it's true that cheetahs could catch us with ease. It would also not be wise to place a wager on a human at a horse race. Humans could however, run down both of these animals over a long distance until their hearts exploded, the reason? Sweat! Humans are able to sweat and when this sweat evaporates, our overall body temperature is cooled.

Many people hate sweating but I embrace this vital trait. Sweat lets me know that I'm exerting myself in an effective way and burning calories. Imagine if primitive humans behaved in the ways that the average person behaves today. Lying around in caves, entertaining themselves with futile activities. We would have never made it out of that era and likely gone extinct if that was the case. The reason that didn't happen was all due to a lack of choice. There were no TV's, cell phones, iPods or distractions of the like. There were only the priorities of food, shelter, water and reproduction. If you weren't mentally and physically fit enough you would perish, period.

Choice has quickly become society's enemy and has forever altered our priorities. Distractions have become so normalized that people forget what's important. It should be abundantly clear that we are not genetically designed to be sedentary all day. Your body doesn't release endorphins if you beat a video game or finish a season of Breaking Bad. Endorphins are hormones secreted within the nervous system and the brain that activate our body's opiate receptors. They are released under moments of stress, pain (like repeated exercise), and extreme pleasure (like sex). I think of Endorphins as a natural reward for doing something that will increase your chances of survival. Think about it; if sex didn't feel so good I guarantee we would have a less populated planet.

If you don't make time for physical activity in your life, you either will or currently are feeling the consequences. I think that if you trap and suppress your physical needs, your body has a tendency to "short circuit" and fulfill this physical need in other ways, such as violence or forced drama in your life. I wish I could do an experiment on every person on earth who suffers from depression, or who is just generally unhappy. I bet a large majority of these people do not exercise and I bet that if they did, many of them would throw their prescriptions out the window.

I'm not trying to discount mental illness in any way. I acknowledge that there are a lot of people who desperately need medication in order to function, due to major chemical imbalances in their brain. My point is that in some cases, people's feelings of emotional imbalance could be fixed or ameliorated through greater fitness levels.

Let's stop lying to ourselves, I mean who doesn't want to look into a mirror and say, "damn, I look great and all my hard work is paying off?" That's an awesome feeling to desire and I think we all should. Break your monotonous cycle and make room for your own fitness. Not only will you look better, but I guarantee you will feel more mentally and physically balanced as well.

If I have a difficult decision to make in my life, if I'm frustrated about something or if I just need some moving meditation, I go for a run or a swim and it helps immensely. I think there's something hypnotic about continuous movement. The ability to feel control over your entire body allows you to transfer this feeling of control to issues within your life.

The purpose of this book is to disclose some of the things that I think can lead to a life of increased fitness. While there is some external research cited, most of the writing here is my opinion or personal experiences of things that work for me. Fitness is more than just a Monday chest day, Tuesday leg day, etc. There are 8 aspects of fitness that I believe people can improve upon to make themselves happier. These 8 aspects are; diet, sleep, flexibility, cardiovascular training, core, functional strength, sex and mental acuity. I will provide only information that I deem to be useful in order to keep things concise. At times I provide opinions from a strictly male perspective, this is not to scare off female readers, it's simply personal experience.

Keep in mind; once you habitually do something, even something painful or difficult, it becomes extraordinarily simple.

"When our physical health is good, we take pleasure in physical exercise, and when our mental health is good, we take pleasure in mental exercise"
-Simon Blackburn

Chapter 2- Diet:

If you eat badly, you will feel badly. This is the most basic yet true statement in the fitness world. If you're going to ignore your eating habits completely and strictly focus on exercise, don't bother reading any further. If you want a great physique you need to eat well, period. Modern society is not designed to aid you in your quest of healthy eating; it is designed to make things that are cheap and convenient for you so that you buy lots. I recently looked up McDonalds health facts; we all know that this sad excuse for a restaurant is bad, but did you know the double quarter pounder meal has almost 3 grams of trans fat? That should be illegal but it's not, why? Because McDonalds is a billion dollar, genius company that knows how to make people buy horrible food for the sake of convenience.

The bottom line here is that you need to take responsibility for your own diet. Do not read the word diet and think 'temporary.' Show me someone on a temporary diet and I'll show you someone who will soon be eating like crap again. Your diet should be your lifestyle; you should make eating well a lifelong habit instead of a two-week fad.

Since there is no universally agreed upon 'perfect diet' I will provide a brief summary of my diet and the rules I try to follow.

-What I Try to Avoid:

Fried foods, white rice, bread, potatoes, cereal, beer/ liquid carbs, fatty sauces, trans fats (obviously), high fructose corn syrup (glucose-fructose in Canada).

* I consume every single thing listed above; I just try to consume very minimal amounts of each.

-What I Typically Try to Eat:

Quinoa & quinoa pasta, whole grain or multigrain bread (if I eat bread at all), avocadoes, kale, spinach, max 2-3 eggs a day, brown rice, ground flaxseed (frozen or refrigerated), chia seeds (great mixed with water), chicken breast, ground tomatoes (substitute for pasta sauce), bananas, natural peanut/ almond butter, dates, unsalted nuts and almonds, black beans, cliff bars, mixed vegetables, unsweetened almond milk, unsweetened coconut water/ oil, LOTS AND LOTS OF WATER!

-Here is what I would consider a good day of eating for myself.

Breakfast:

Large smoothie consisting of 1 banana, 4 dates, 1 tbs of natural peanut butter, 1 handful or kale/ spinach, 1 tbs of ground flaxseed, 1 tbs of chia seeds, 1 tbs of coconut oil, 1 tbs of honey, lots of cinnamon, 1 handful of assorted frozen fruit, unsweetened almond milk and coconut water (add until there's a sufficient amount of liquid in the smoothie.)

Lunch:

Burrito made with whole-wheat pita, avocado, black beans, quinoa/ brown rice, tomatoes, tuna, and sweet potato.

Snack:

Cliff bar, carrots and broccoli.

Dinner:

Chicken quinoa with natural tomato sauce (crushed tomatoes), spinach salad with some light vinaigrette dressing

As you can see, my breakfast packs a punch and I fit as many things as I can into my smoothie. With my smoothies I also take 1000 IU of vitamin D, one Jamieson Vita-vim multivitamin, 1200mg of fish oil, and 1200 mcg of vitamin B12. It's especially important to stay hydrated during the day if you are staying active and sweating. Every time I pass a water fountain I take a drink and I always try to keep a water bottle with me.

Once a week I have a cheat day and I spike my caloric intake by eating whatever I want, which normally means a lot of junk food. Contrary to what you may think, this is not a bad thing and it will allow you to maintain a healthy diet throughout the week. Sometimes if I find I can't wait for one specific day, I will have a couple of cheat meals during the week instead. If 90% of what you're eating is healthy then you're allowed to slip up sometimes.

Keep in mind that I am not a nutritionist or a dietician. This is simply what I tend to eat/ avoid, it works very well for me and I feel awesome when I follow the above guidelines. I have weighed between 180 and 192 pounds for the last seven years. This was only possible because I realized that as my metabolism began to slow, I needed to change my eating habits and continuously exercise in order to not put on weight. Below are two pictures of me; I've never taken a supplement in my entire life, not even a protein shake. These companies want you to get hooked on buying their products so that you feel like you need them to get fit and stay fit, when in reality you do not.

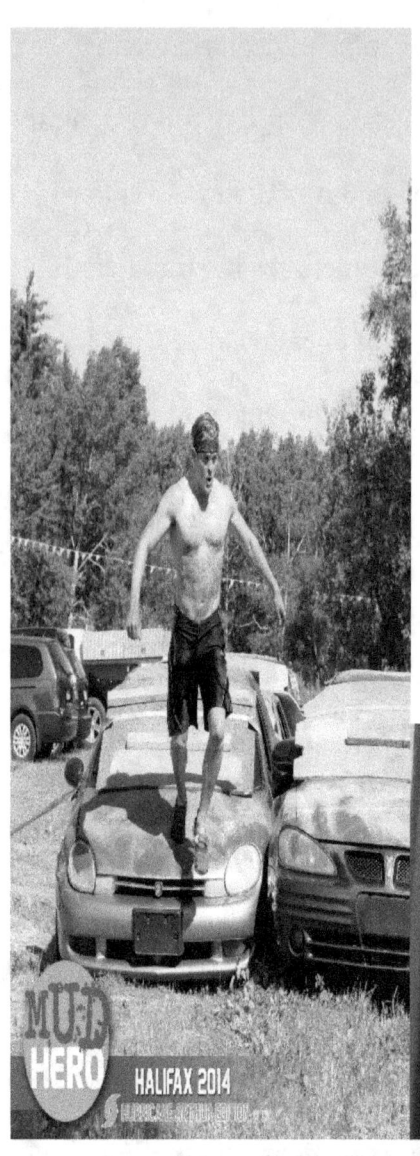

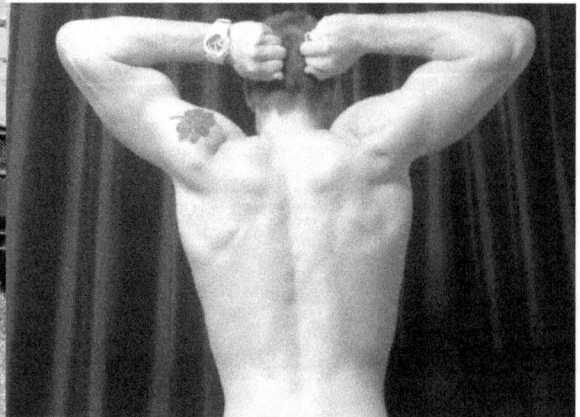

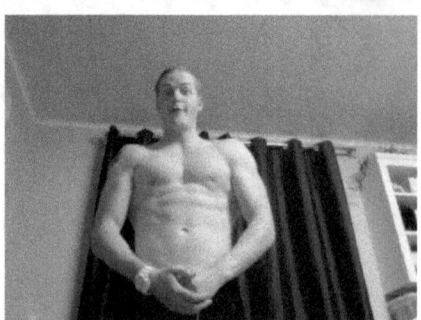

You won't see me on stage at a bodybuilding or physique competition but I don't care, I feel great and I never have to starve or dehydrate myself to win a fake "fitness/ health" title.

Chapter 3- Sleep:

Sleep is obviously a crucial factor when it comes to your energy level. Most people solemnly believe that 8 hours is the universally prescribed sleep duration. Dean Karnazes is a living rebuttal of the 8-hour claim. Karnazes decided that he was wasting too much time sleeping so he began sleeping 4 hours a night. This seems to be working for him because he regularly competes in ultra marathons and he once ran 50 consecutive marathons, in all 50 of the United States, in 50 days, all on 4 hours of sleep per night. This guy is obviously a freak of nature when it comes to running, but could he be on to something when it comes to sleep cycles?

I don't claim to sleep 4 hours a night; I usually get between 6 and 7, sometimes with a 20-minute nap during the day. Tim Ferris did extensive research on polyphasic sleep (sleeping multiple times within 24 hours) in "The 4 Hour Body." Ferris essentially found that for every 1.5 hours of core sleep you subtract, you can still feel just as energized if you add a twenty minute nap during the day. These naps should be strict and as close to twenty minutes as you can possibly get. I personally find Ferris' model to work, but only to a certain extent. Once you dip below 3 hours of core sleep and 3 twenty-minute naps, things begin to get a little iffy. I do not know anybody who has time for 5 or 6 naps during the day and I found it impossible to stay energized running on anything less than 3 hours of core sleep. Even 3 hours of core sleep with 3 naps sometimes left me feeling exhausted.

One thing Ferris definitely gets wrong in his book is sleep position. He claims that sleeping on your stomach; in an immobilizing half military crawl position, is the best way to sleep. If you don't have a spine or if you're immune to back pain then this position might work for you. Otherwise, you should sleep on your back with pillow(s) under your knees, or you could do your back an even bigger favor and sleep on your side, with one pillow between your legs, one under your head and one under the arm that's on top. I try to use the latter sleeping position as much as possible, especially since I injured my back a few years ago. Every chiropractor, physiotherapist and Osteopath I went to recommended this position, and I have to say it works very well.

I would advise you to question the 8-hour sleep model and play around with different core sleeping and nap schedules. You might find that you can give yourself more productive time in exchange for less sleep, all while maintaining similar or higher energy levels. I try not to eat within an hour of going to sleep to avoid putting on weight and I try to stick to a consistent sleeping position as much as possible. As juvenile as it sounds, setting a bedtime is a great idea. When I'm traveling on a budget, camping every night, I tend to sleep when it gets dark and rise at first light. This is a great, but difficult routine to keep. I find sleeping in too much is never a great idea, as it personally leaves me feeling sluggish and tired for the rest of the day.

Chapter 4- Flexibility:

This is my weakest area of fitness, so I write this chapter as someone trying to gain better flexibility by experimenting with new techniques. I remember being forced to stretch in gym class throughout school when I was younger and hating every second of it. Most people, when they are young, are so flexible that they take that level of flexibility for granted. I used to be flexible, then I competed as a kayaker for 7 years, not stretching nearly enough, and now I am as inflexible as a rusty robot.

My downfall was not doing post-workout stretching. I almost never stretched after I had done either a vigorous kayaking or weight workout. I would just leave the paddling club with super tense muscles, head home and go to sleep. Years of this routine have certainly taken a toll on me and I've faced my fair share of injuries because of it.

By increasing your flexibility, you can increase the range of motion for any exercise that you do. Getting full range of motion is very important if you want to get the most out of every single rep that you do. Quality always beats quantity when it comes to working out. Before doing any of the exercises in this book, make sure you start slow and learn the proper techniques first. If there's weight involved in the exercise you should always start light!

Since incorporating proper warm-ups before my workouts and at least 15 minutes of post- workout stretching I have yet to get another injury. I used to stretch before my workouts but now I only stretch afterwards. This is because I was getting injured about once a year from lifting weights. Two sports therapists suggested that I switch my stretching to after my workout and do dynamic warm-ups at the beginning of workouts. I took this advice and it has been working very well for me. Here are some good dynamic warm-ups:

Warm-up A) 5- 10 minutes of skipping, 20 lunges

Warm-up B) 30 arms circles (15 each way), 5 burpees, 20 squats, 20 jumping jacks

Warm-up C) 2 X 30 reps of: jumping jacks, high knees, seal jacks

These don't have to be difficult, just something to get you moving before your main workout. After your main workout you should stretch for 15- 20 minutes. Not only will this aid your worked muscles in recovering, but you will also be less sore the next day. Daily stretching sessions will increase flexibility tremendously and decrease the likelihood of getting injured in the gym.

I have sometimes entered the gym feeling slow, weak and sluggish and cancelled my workouts in order to stretch for 40 minutes. On these days I always leave the gym feeling much better than I did coming in. If you come to the realization that you're too tired to get anything out of a scheduled workout, don't feel bad about stretching instead because this is still productive in the long run. I give myself one day completely off in my workout schedule, so I try to stretch lots on that day as well. There are tons of examples of some great stretches for different muscles online. Search 'Mayo clinic guide to basic stretches' on Google for a good starting point. Try to create your own stretching routine and stick to it everyday. I try to hold every single stretch that I do for at least thirty seconds. Make sure you don't over stretch though because this can damage your muscles; I do about 18 different stretches for thirty seconds each and that's it. If you stretch every day for two weeks you will definitely notice an increase in flexibility. Foam rollers are another great way to loosen up your muscles before or after a workout. I tend to use a foam roller after my workouts are complete.

Another way I was able to dramatically increase my flexibility was participating in Brazilian jiu jitsu. This low impact martial art forces you to become flexible in order to survive. You're forced to contort your body in many different ways in order to not tap out and lose matches. Two or three weeks of hard jiu jitsu training and you're sure to notice a difference in flexibility. Flexibility isn't the only benefit of jiu jitsu, it's also an amazing full- body workout and you will learn things like how to control your breathing, how to channel your anger, applicable self-defense skills, and how to keep your ego in check.

Chapter 5- Core:

This is my absolute favorite part of working out. Prepare yourself for some core workouts from hell! The core is the essence of your entire body and if your core is weak, you are weak. Keep in mind that your core is more than just your abs; it is the stabilization system of your entire body. I find that when I'm working my core a lot, my general workout techniques tend to improve, I feel more balanced and I'm way less likely to get an injury. I work my core at least 3 times a week and the stronger my core gets, the more I enjoy the gym.

Doing ab workouts is not going to get you a six-pack, unless you eat well and have no belly fat. If you have an awful diet and a lot of belly fat, it doesn't matter how hard you work your abs because the fat will be covering the results. You have to burn that fat off by doing intense core and cardio workouts.

I never lie on my back for twenty minutes and work my abs, I like to get more of my core involved because it's more fun and productive. I will now provide some core circuit workouts that I often do. I will only explain an exercise if I don't think you would be able to find it on the Internet. Every workout is circuit style with one-minute rest upon completion of a full set, no rest between exercises! The circuit style ads a cardio aspect to the workouts, making them all the more challenging. Remember, and this going for all workouts, once you feel the burn KEEP GOING! If you give up as soon as you feel the pain, then you are wasting the crucial moments of your workouts.

Workout A) 3 Sets of: 30 seconds flexed arm hang (hanging onto chin-up bar at eye level with arms bent), 25 Russian twists, 30 Kettle bell swings @ 40 lbs, 25 leg lifts, 1:30 plank, 50 air squats.

Workout B) 4 X 10-15 Reps each of: burpees , muscle ups (10- 15 reps, or until failure), lunges, TRX pikes, mountain climbers, squat jumps, bicycles, sit ups.

Workout C) 1 Minute of each exercise, 2 minutes rest, 1 minute of each exercise: speed skaters, burpees, plank, kettle bell Turkish getups, leg over's, flexed arm hang, penguins, mountain climbers, flutter kicks.

Workout D) 5 Sets of: 100 double unders (skipping), 30 burpees.

There you have it, some core workouts that are sure to burn! If you get bored of certain workouts it's easy to mix up the exercises and create your own, it's actually really fun once you get good at it. The hard part is determining if the workout will be too easy or too difficult. When I'm writing workouts I often forget that I'm not a superhuman, and that fatigue is a real thing that is out to get me. When I started writing my own workouts I had to practice writing realistic and manageable sets, but now I've pretty much worked out (no pun intended) all the bugs. If you find these workouts too tough or too easy, you can always increase or decrease the sets and/ or reps and weight.

Chapter 6- Cardiovascular Training:

When you hear cardiovascular training please don't picture a treadmill. I never use treadmills and I think they are torture. My favorite form of cardio is swimming and I try to get into the pool at least twice a week. Swimming is difficult to get decent at if you're a beginner but once you get the hang of it, you'll never look back. In order to make swimming a good cardio workout you need to do it for a fair amount of time. I aim for thirty minutes to one hour per workout. Once you're able to relax in the pool and swim effortlessly, I find it to be a rather hypnotizing activity. I often swim for hundreds of meters without even realizing how far I've gone.

There's something about the quietness under the water that allows you to enter a kind of meditative state. I do some of my best thinking when I'm submerged in the pool doing a workout. The best way to get better at swimming (focus on front crawl) is to watch online technique videos, get somebody to take a video of you swimming so you can compare techniques. I recommend doing lots of flutter kick and lots of strokes with a pull buoy. Understanding how to coordinate your arms with your legs is difficult to do; I try to kick three times for every one stroke that I take. As far as breathing goes I try to breathe every 2 strokes, then 3 and then 2 so that the side I breathe on is being alternated.

Running is obviously what most people view as the epitome of cardio training. Many people find running boring but that's likely because they're not having fun with it. I find trail running to be very fun and I also think running on the street is fun if you challenge yourself. I like to use a GPS and measure the distance of my runs, whether it is a 2km, 6km or 10km run, etc. Once I have a variety of different distances, I time myself to try to improve my time in all distances. Striving to better your times when you run is very rewarding, and learning how to compete with yourself is crucial if you're usually working out on your own.

As far as running goes, the book "Born to Run" by Christopher McDougall has some great information in it. McDougall observes the behavior of elite Mexican running tribes and essentially finds that the key to running injury free is to keep your weight on the balls of your feet and not to slam down onto the cushioned heels of the running shoes. Your feet are designed to act as shock absorbers, and by slamming onto your heels you defeat the purpose of this design. He also suggests implementing some barefoot running into your schedule in order to strengthen your feet, which are always pampered with shoes, and to force yourself to run on the balls of your feet. I try to force myself to run on my toes and take shorter, faster steps. I followed these tips and within days, the lower back pain I normally experience while running was eliminated, and I took my 10km time down from 41:11 to 38:57.

McDougall also looks into the benefits of chia seeds. He finds that one of the keys to the Mexican runners dominance, is that fact that they eat chia seeds for quick energy during their runs. I now mix chia seeds into my water when I run. They are flavorless with a subtle texture, an amazing source of protein and omega 3's. I can genuinely say that I do feel more energized when I drink these seeds when I run and I recommend trying it.

Indoor rowing machines also offer a fantastic cardio workout. I only really got into rowing this year, but so far I'm enjoying it a lot. Doing a 500-meter row as fast as you can is a great indication of how you're doing. By doing some of the following workouts and focusing on proper technique, I was able to take my 500-meter time down from 1:41 to 1:23. This was a difficult feat, one that I'm quite proud of. Here are some of my favorite workouts.

Workout A) 3 x 500m row with 30 Kettlebell swings (40lbs) in between each set.

Workout B) 2 minutes easy rowing, 1 minute hard rowing X 8

Workout C) 4 x 500m row with one-minute rest between sets. Aim to see how low you can get your average 500m time

More than any aspect of fitness, I find that cardio is the main branch for improving the way your body feels in general. When I have been running a lot I almost feel as though the resistance of gravity has been slightly decreased. I feel more spring in my step; I can get around faster, float up staircases and never seem to get fatigued in day-to-day life.

The feeling of having good cardio is spectacular, and the endorphin rush you feel after completing a good workout is fantastic. Don't get caught in the mind-set that cardio needs to be an extremely time consuming activity. While I do enjoy long cardio workouts, I often cut them back to 20-30 minutes if I'm on a time constraint. Cardio and functional strength workouts compliment each other nicely. If you're doing something like kettle bells or a weight circuit for a long time, make no mistake that you are also getting in a great cardio workout.

Chapter 7- Functional Strength:

Functional strength is the kind of strength that will aid you in your day-to-day tasks. Examples are; lifting and moving heavy objects, completing tasks without losing as much energy, and just having more all-around full body strength. If you have a lot of functional strength you will feel more connected to your entire body and you will be able to operate as one complete unit. Instead of having strong legs but a weak back, or a powerful chest with a feeble core, functional strength will allow you to gain an overall sense of power throughout your entire body.

If you can bench press 300 pounds with proper form, that's good, but it doesn't necessarily mean you have functional strength. In the course of a day how often do you have to lie horizontally and press weight completely vertically? Do you see my point? Functional strength will allow you to perform realistic tasks with minimal fatigue and maximum efficiency.

Enough talk, lets get down to some exercises that will give you functional strength. Kettle bells are the pinnacle of functional strength. Originating in Russia these awesome fitness tools have recently been popularized in North America. I bought a 40-pound kettle bell this year and it's the best fitness investment I've ever made. Some of my favorite kettle bell exercises are the two handed swing, snatch, up-right row with a squat, slingshot, halo and Turkish getup. As previously mentioned, if done correctly kettle bells are a great cardio workout. Even if you do a few sets, two minutes each for the exercises above, you will understand what I mean.

I find that the hanging pull-up and the burpee are two other gems of functional strength. By hanging pull-up I mean that there is no kip/swing involved, you're simply pulling your chin straight up over the bar. Focus on quality reps, not quantity. For burpees make sure you are getting your chest right down to the ground and jumping straight up at the end of each rep. Battle rope swings are also a great exercise if you feel like enduring some pain.

I really enjoy these two workouts, which involve some of what I just talked about:

Workout A) 3 pull ups, 3 burpees, 10 kettle bells swings, 2 Turkish getups

5 pull ups, 5 burpees, 15 kettle bell swings, 4 Turkish getups

10 pull ups, 10 burpees, 30 kettle bell swings, 8 turkish getups.

X 2 or 3

Workout B) 1:00 on, 1:00 off, 45 seconds on of each exercise:

Push ups, kettle bell sling shots, burpees, kettle bell swings, jumping jacks, pull ups, kettle bell upright row with squat, mountain climbers, kettle bell snatches, Turkish getups, up & down battle rope swings.

If you can increase your functional strength, then you will increase your everyday efficiency. Workouts like these often garner strange looks at the gym, simply because they are not in the average persons exercise repertoire. It doesn't matter; these people don't know what they're missing, so just do your thing!

"I put myself into a mind state where it feels like I'm about to fight for my life. The mindset you take into working out is very important. The reality of the situation is, the more intense you are, the more effort you put into the workout, the more explosion you bring to the workout, the more you're going to get out of it, and that's just a fact."
-Joe Rogan

Chapter 8- The Benefits of Sex:

Being a qualified sex expert I will attempt to......

No, that's a lie. I have no great secrets; all I know is that there is no better post workout activity than sex, obviously. A big part of the reason that people want to be fit is so that they can attract a mate who will want to have sex with them regularly. I know this is all very mind blowing, but stay with me.

I can think of no greater reward for being fit than the fact that you will likely have more sex. A greater sense of wellbeing is clearly the best reward, but sex is part of that greater wellbeing! Sex keeps your body and mind in check, and without it things start to get unbalanced.

The only real secret that I use while having sex is the way I breathe. By being able to control your breathing the whole way through, you enable yourself to last longer. I didn't believe this when I read it in "The Multi-Orgasmic Couple," but the next time I had sex I realized how frantic my breathing was as I neared the end of my session. I began to breathe in a slow steady pattern and I was able to control myself. As I practiced this breathing technique I continued to get better and better. It's harder than it sounds because your breathing is so out of sync with the motion of your body, but it becomes easy after a while. Just remember to focus on diaphragmatic breathing (deep belly breathing) and keeping a slow steady breathing pattern (Abrams & Chia).

Having a consistent sex partner whom you feel comfortable communicating and trying new things with, is crucial for the betterment of your sexual skill. Don't be afraid to ask questions and make suggestions with your partner. It's important to find out what one another likes best, so that you can both have the most pleasurable experience possible.

As I previously mentioned, Brazilian jiu jitsu is a great way to learn how to control your breathing. Not to mention that it also strengthens your body in ways that are conducive to better, less fatigued sex.

Chapter 9- Mental Acuity:

Mental discipline is crucial when doing long, painful workouts. I often have to mentally prepare for a while before beginning a long workout or a difficult exercise set. If your head isn't in the game you won't perform to your full potential. Don't start a workout unless you're mentally prepared to endure some pain!

Your brain is a tool and it must be worked constantly in order to stay strong. I don't feel 100% unless I've physically and mentally exerted myself. Read a book, watch some VICE news videos or have some meaningful, in depth conversations with friends. I think this last one is very important. If you only have friends who want to talk about getting drunk and the drama in their lives, maybe it's time to get some new ones. Every once in a while it's super refreshing to have deep conversations.

Conversations about current events, the meaning of life, the universe or maybe the fact that we're all just on a rock, surviving because we are orbiting a massive fireball, wandering around on this lonely planet, completely confused.

One of my favorite sources of current information is the Joe Rogan Experience Podcast. Not only is this podcast hilarious, but extremely informative. Rogan interviews a myriad of different guests, all bringing unique information and viewpoints to the table. Rogan is able to keep an open mind and he asks some of the most intelligent questions you can imagine. Throughout the years this podcast has evolved from a basement joke session to a more professional, but not too professional, interview atmosphere. I don't even listen to music on my iPod anymore because it's just the same repetitive stuff. I'd rather learn something when I'm bored enough to put my headphones in.

One of my favorite pastimes is watching stand-up comedy. This brilliant art form is quite amazing when done correctly. Comedians are granted a unique immunity when they take center stage. Just by being present, the audience has agreed that they will let the comedian openly speak their mind. The fact that the comedian can say whatever they want and not be taken seriously is awesome. This allows the comedian to discuss any matter they please with total immunity, and often times their deeper message still gets through to the crowd. I enjoy comedians who question the norms of society and force people to rethink their ideals. Some of my favorites, in no particular order are Bill Burr, Joe Rogan, Duncan Trussell, Chris Rock, Dave Chapelle and Patrice O'neal.

Never be afraid to look dumb or you will never learn. Ask questions until you find out exactly what you want to know. Your ego is your enemy; don't let it ruin you because once you stop learning, you become arrogant and irrelevant.

"The mind always fails first, not the body. The secret is to make your mind work for you, not against you."
-Arnold Schwarzenegger

Chapter 10- Conclusion:

In conclusion, this book is merely a representation of my own personal experiences and the guidelines I try to follow in order to become a more happy and productive person. Everything I said is exactly what I do because it works very well for me, but this is not to say that it will work for you.

Hopefully this book will serve as your brief, yet difficult guide to a greater level of general fitness. Allow me to reiterate: fitness is not a simple thing to achieve or maintain and anybody who tells you otherwise is lying to you, likely to make a quick buck. Fitness must be achieved, maintained and constantly improved upon. It is a lifestyle choice that will make you a happier person. You only have one body, so try to make it the best physical specimen that you possibly can

Pardon yet another car analogy but I find it ironic that some people spend their entire lives saving up for dream cars. They feel that if they can just afford that Ferrari, they will be a complete and happy person. People will go into debt to buy a nice car, yet throw their own personal well being on the back burner. Invest your money in something natural and real, like your body. I bet a woman would find a healthy guy in a Honda to be more attractive than a fat-ass in a Ferrari. All I know is that I'd rather feel good in my own body than in a luxury car, but I'm obviously going to strive to be fit and also drive a badass car.

Never give your body a simple solution or let it get comfortable. Always keep your body guessing so it's able to do what it does best; adapt to the most adverse and arduous of circumstances.

-John Mayo

Bibliography

Abrams & Chia. *The Multi-Orgasmic Couple*. New York: Harper Collins

Publishers,   2002. Print.

Blackburn, Simon. *Think*. New York: Oxford University Press, 1999. Print

Ferris, Timothy. *The 4-Hour Body: An Uncommon Guide to Rapid Fat-*

Loss, Incredible   *Sex, and Becoming Superhuman.*

Crown Publishing Group, 2010. Print.

McDougall, Christopher. *Born to Run: A Hidden Tribe, Superathletes and*

the greatest   *Race the World has Never*

Seen. New York: Alfred A. Knopf, 2009. Print.